WORK, WORKOUT & MORE

A MINIMALISTIC & REALISTIC APPROACH OF BODYBUILDING AND FITNESS FOR "BUSY" PROFESSIONALS.

SANDIPAN HALDAR

Copyright © Sandipan Haldar
All Rights Reserved.

This book has been published with all efforts taken to make the material error-free after the consent of the author. However, the author and the publisher do not assume and hereby disclaim any liability to any party for any loss, damage, or disruption caused by errors or omissions, whether such errors or omissions result from negligence, accident, or any other cause.

While every effort has been made to avoid any mistake or omission, this publication is being sold on the condition and understanding that neither the author nor the publishers or printers would be liable in any manner to any person by reason of any mistake or omission in this publication or for any action taken or omitted to be taken or advice rendered or accepted on the basis of this work. For any defect in printing or binding the publishers will be liable only to replace the defective copy by another copy of this work then available.

This book is dedicated to every person in the world who deserve to lead a good healthy life on their own way.

Contents

Foreword

Fitness is a word that needs no introduction in this current time that's true, but you all will agree to the fact that it takes a little bit extra push to get into this habit. Specially at this time while writing the book when the entire human race is going through a tumultuous phase due the covid-19 pandemic, we all must have murmured to us to promote ourselves into the fitness journey. Having said that, it's not about only for this time being, it's about the lifestyle you choose over a long period of time to remain motivated and happy.

From my very own experience and interaction with several people over the years, I have observed how difficult it is to maintain a fitness routine over long period of time when you are someone working 8-12 hours daily behind the desk. There are lot of aspects actually which emphasizes the word "difficult" here. Sometime we blame it to our working schedules, our own time mismanagement, being not too encouraged, overly lazy or most importantly not too practical in our fitness goals. I am pretty sure, whoever is struggling to be consistent in this path must have come across the reasons I just mentioned earlier. Also, it is needless to say that in our current lifestyle, getting time to dig in through different materials is very difficult. Over the years I always tried to know the right approaches, right techniques about the fitness. So, I googled a lot over different authentic articles, watched lot of you tube videos of many experts in this profession just to gather as much knowledge as I can.

Here in this book, I have tried to collate all those knowledges in simple words just to ease that process for you. So, through this book I want to show some way to get out of those difficulties and happily sail through your fitness dreams. I also have tried to pinpoint the mistakes to avoid for you people which I have faced over these years. All I need from you people is to *believe in the process* and if I can do then it is pretty much doable for all of you as well.

First of all, I wanted to say that I am not a geek from the fitness industry to walk you through all the niches of fitness. So, I don't want to blabber lot of fancy jargons here through this book just to confuse you. Now a days, there are mundane of information out there in the internet which can easily overwhelm you just to become perplexed. But I am here to help you achieve your smallest wish/goals in terms of fitness, through this book. Working towards your goal calls for some patience from your side which you must possess. If not right after you complete reading this book, but sometime later in your life you will definitely thank me even in your back of the mind. I am very much confident about that. With the small tricks and methods, I have explained, you can certainly become the best version of yourself. So, let's keep it short and crisp for now and assist you further. As part of a little *disclaimer* is, may be since I am little inclined to weight training & muscle building, in this book I have emphasized more on that side. But in reality, the ideas are very much applicable for any form of fitness someone is attributed to.

Acknowledgements

I would like to thank my parents, my wife and my friends a lot, who has appreciated my dedication to fitness over the years. That is one of the reason i really wanted to share my stories that can help so many people out there to achieve their desired bodies.

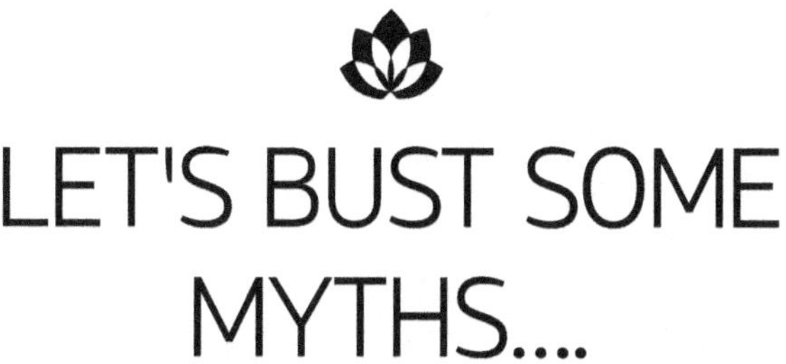

LET'S BUST SOME MYTHS....

Life on Social Media

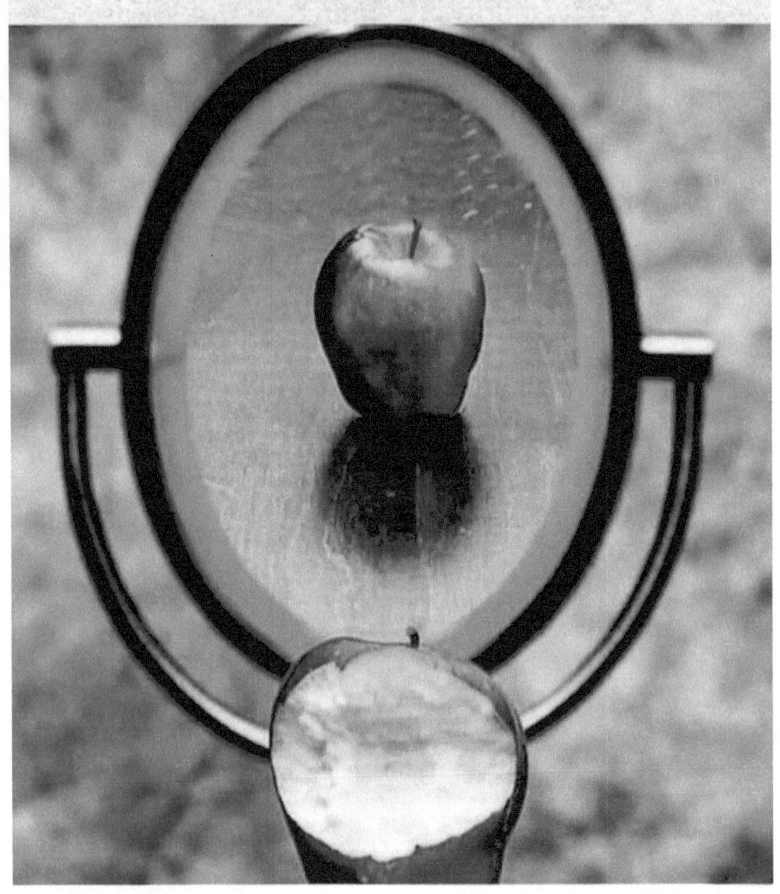

Life On Social Media

To begin with the discussion about this crucial topic, I really want you people to understand the meaning of the above pic. Scrolling through my Instagram feed, I saw this one day and I just found it so apt to explain few points here.

You might see lot of Instagram, you tube influencers are sharing their knowledges day in day out. But trust me not all of them are telling you the truth. People get easily carried away with few headings like "abs in 30 days", "fat loss in 1 week", "1-inch biceps addition in one month" and so on. These are extremely misguiding and you have to accept the fact wholeheartedly. And most of the people (not all of them) are just exploiting these platforms like this. So, it is very important that we understand the ground reality first. We need to be very practical when it comes to our goals, fitness is no exception. Most of the times, being carried away with the claims from you tube videos/Instagram, people just don't see their results and then get frustrated and leave the journey very soon. Very few eminent personalities you will see who really speaks the truth when it comes to share their fitness knowledge.

I am going to give you some heads-up about the *common myths* about bodybuilding which keep on circulating from time immemorial. You should take note of these, even if you feel to experience your own then please go ahead and understand yourself. I am just making you people aware of these beforehand so that you can avoid digging them in the hard way.

a. *CARBs are very bad for health*:

This is one of the greatest myths you will ever come across from a fellow gym goer these days. The main reason behind this is the ignorance and not fully aware of the exact theory. Carbs are definitely needed for your body to grow, otherwise you will just run out of energy and may not be able to work to your full potential. It's all about the calorie intake and burning that defines whether you are going towards weight gain or weight loss. For example, if some lean person is trying to put on some muscle as per his goal and then he comes to know this myth and keep on maintaining the same for years he is definitely not going to see the minimum of results of his hard work. Idea is to have caloric surplus when someone is trying to gain weight and to be in caloric deficit when someone is trying to lose weight. It is really that simple as you heard my friend. The entire game is between calorie intake and burn, it is your job to keep it simple like this. So, remember, carbs are not your enemy.

a. ***Doing countless crunches to get the abs:***

If you want your abs to be visible then foremost thing you need to take care is to check your caloric intake. The spot reduction of body fats doesn't happen for real. Overall staying in caloric deficit together with few abs' exercises will ensure those abs are visible. Diet is the main focus here.

c. ***The influencers/actors are always jacked:***

Most of the times when we watch any movies or some videos of some influencers in the social media, we feel that how they maintain their body to be jacked and pumped always. Even I also wondered for long time. You might think your pump is just gone in a day or so. Basically, the truth is, before every shoot they do some pumping exercises to make their muscles look prominent in front of the camera. And that's the ask of their profession. So, for us normal people we don't have to be just get discouraged or confused. You might have noticed few actors/bodybuilders also in some casual interviews, where they don't look like what you saw previously in photos as totally ripped. Even the professional bodybuilders who comes on stage shows, they have to do lot of pumping exercises before that. Also, you need to understand one more thing, there are few anabolic, steroid which some people use as part of their profession as well. But we absolutely don't need this in our goal. So, all I am trying to repeat is to have a very practical mindset when you are through this process of your bodybuilding journey. Don't compare yourself with anybody. You might be unable to workout for a month and see somebody else looking muscular than you, and suddenly you hurry up on some workout moves afterwards just to make yourself uncomfortable and ultimately keeping yourself out of action for some more time.

d. ***You need to do more repetitions when you are in weight loss regime*:**

This is also one more misunderstood topic I would say. You really can follow your weight loss regime by lifting heavy weight and doing standard rep sets as well. Lifting heavy itself will ensure more work over the resistance and more calories being burnt. So, it is not any hard and fast rule to go with only higher repetitions.

e. ***You need to work out every day to grow fast*:**

The principle of muscle growth is you need to have ample rest throughout the week considering your workout days. Muscle only grows when it is not working. So, its outside the gym when the muscle is grown. Proper diet, sleep etc. are all is needed for better results. You have to remember that 'less is more' when it comes to muscle building progress. You need to *scientifically* follow the process and everything else will take care of itself.

The aforementioned points are just few of many **myths going round the fitness industries** these days. I personally faced these queries also from my colleagues in the gym. Probably believing those myths led them to stop hitting gym after some days. So, I urge you honestly to be very aware and very much knowledgeable while following the process.

"*The Road to nowhere is paved with excuses.*" – Mark Bell, World record holding professional powerlifter & fitness coach.

CHAPTER TWO

WHEN, WHERE AND HOW?...

Ok, as you read through the title of this chapter you are 100% sure that the answers are very simple enough to guess. As the saying goes, the good time to start was *'yesterday'* and the next good time is *'today'*, and you can start anywhere with anything you feel compatible with your workout session. But the hurdles everyone (including me) faces are the lethargy, excuses, challenges in our everyday professional and personal lives. I must say these are some real reasons to deal with except the word "excuse".

Over the next few paragraphs, I want to share my own way to handle these obstacles from the start of my own fitness journey back in 2013 during my MTECH days in IIT Bombay. For me it was the vibe of staying in Mumbai that triggered my inner feeling to jump into bodybuilding. Working out for few days gave me a good feeling overall which I *chose* to continue for some more days, and then it became a habit. Before that while in college days, I was very active playing outdoor games almost regularly. I used to be a very lean guy from the time I was kid. But one day I decided to make it happen when I entered into the hostel gym to do weight training for the first time. To be honest that day changed my life forever and also that day has paved the way to gather courage to write this book as a naive writer, so that it can help many of you out there fulfill your long wish to looks good physically.

It will be a blatant lie if none of us confess now, that you never wished to have a great muscular physique while you bumped onto some pictures of the ripped Bollywood actors or a Schwarzenegger or seeing a guy in the road having a better body than you. Now if you are honest enough to agree with me about the above fact, then trust me I will certainly assist you to make your dream come true to certain extent (rest will be your wish). I am not going to tell you about some specific workout routines or any fad diets to follow in this book, as you know there are plethora of books, experts, YouTube videos, articles and so on. I am neither a professional in bodybuilding nor I did some bodybuilding courses to be a trainer. But you can consider me as your mental trainer who will change your physique forever.

While in the hostel during my MTech, almost every day whenever I got some spare time, I used to surf around all the different bodybuilding articles and learn from them. It is true that, at that point of time I was new to it so it must be out of bubbling enthusiasm I did that, but the fact is even today I try to learn about it, about the same old workout to get into perfection. And in my opinion, that's what matters most. It's the consistency that will help you achieve your goal even in this field. The body that you are looking for or licking your lips seeing someone out there with a good physique, you can also reach but you just need to keep in mind that it's a marathon race not to think about outright result. This much you need to train your mind to achieve the physical greatness. I encourage you to start it today and dig deep to learn the right techniques of your workouts. Don't go for some fancy stuffs you come across almost every day on you tubes and end up losing your gas and confused. Always think it about a long-time investment on yourself. If you are consistent enough in initial few years you will get to see the results quick enough which must give you more Viagra to stick to it. But one word of caution is, don't get blown away with the term "quick", it is very overrated I must say.

There are so many generous people out there in fitness industry, who share lots of workout routines, which are easily available on the internet. Just go there, research a bit and stick to it. You have to do this part on your own. But there will also be a state of confusion as I myself experienced, when you try to gasp all those knowledges. But don't get confused, don't get overwhelmed at all, just do it step by step, do it consistently. You are not going to take part in some professional competition (unless you change your current career goal) so that you have to take the shortest route. Just think, you are not in a hurry at all.

Now comes the hardest part, the challenge of managing your time. We all faces this challenge differently at every phase of the life. During the MTech days, it was the class timings that used to collide with my own gym timing. And now it is some urgent meetings that will keep you really in a hard place to take time out for your fitness habit. But the solution is you have to find out some or other way. It's not that I haven't missed any of my daily workout routine, you are also bound to miss it. There will be deadlines in your profession as well but the idea is to continue it. You may miss hitting the gym for 7 consecutive days due to your own challenges, but you should keep it at your heart that someday when you get a chance next you will certainly take the opportunity. And this is the secret for your success nothing else, I promise.

Now coming to the point where to start, ideally you can start anywhere. The most important aspect of being consistent in this fitness journey is, you need to be very flexible. What I meant by the word 'flexible' is, you shouldn't think that you cannot start today because you don't have any major gym equipment with you. As we all got very accustomed these days during corona, we tried to be very innovative at our home when it comes to continue the workout. So, my message also will be same to you. Let off your excuses, just wake up from being lazy and do some basic things to move on. Even people who used to have gym membership or access to a gym anyhow, should continue the same in alternate ways at home. Some of us already bought some handy gears as well to do the workout at home. But even if you don't have any, you can always do some bodyweight workouts at your own will. Also coming to the topic again that "we are being so busy in most of the days of week", in that case also if you are already accustomed with decent home workout regime, that should help your cause too in those days. You might feel little tired or lazy (fair enough to be felt like that) going out to hit your outside gym, but the habit you already developed staying at home will certainly help you make a little gain on that day as well. I always feel that being in a disciplined life is more mental. You might be doing some physical workout at the end of the day, but first you need to win the mental battle. Now the point is, you need to train your mind first then the body will definitely follow.

Initial few days might be very tough for you to drown upon this lifestyle, but once you start feeling good and more confident you will definitely want to continue this for life. Investing in yourself is the best thing you can think of at any point of your life and the opportunity has just come now to you. So, without wasting time or confusing yourself let's start your workout with whatever little help you have at your home or your gym.

> Excuses make today easy, but tomorrow hard.
>
> Discipline makes today hard, but tomorrow easy.

#thought

One very important psychological viewpoint I want to discuss here is, don't just be disheartened by small irregularities. I know once you get used to this lifestyle, you might find it very difficult at some phase of the year for whatever real reasons it might be.

You might think your gains are going to fade etc. but trust me when you focus on discipline and continuity everything falls back to a place again. Also, we have to be very practical in our thinking as well. The pictures you see even for some Bollywood actors in social media or anywhere, you don't need to believe all those to be honest. When you do it naturally, you are not supposed to be looked fully pumped and muscular always. So don't just let yourself down or overthink how those people are always looked so ripped. Even they come for photoshoot after significant pumping and yes that's the truth. Basically, as the saying goes by just try improving your physique only considering yourself as the competitor nobody else. Being realistic in your goal means a lot in this fitness journey. Always think it as a long-term investment on yourself. There is no meaning of getting the coveted x-pack abs with 6-12 months of hard work and then stay unfit for life.

"Victory isn't defined by wins and losses, it's defined by effort." – **Kai Greene, IFBB Professional Bodybuilder**

CHAPTER THREE

THE FLEXIBLE WORKOUT ROUTINE

Now that all the motivations you may have got already, it's time to make it feasible. I am very careful on the word 'feasible' here, I really want to emphasize on it and want to tell you something that is very much practical to follow, given all the worldly commitments you have throughout the days, months and years.

We should understand first the value of a routine. It actually means a discipline which we follow (rather should follow) at every aspect of our lives, to make it a part of our lives. Let's be very honest here, we are very obsessed with the word 'motivation', isn't it? But trust me, motivation has its expiry so what to do then? You will feel like having excuses to avoid doing workout then (it happens even if you are very regular in your workout regime). So, at that moment, discipline will carry you forward to break the shackles. Basically, it is a mixture of both motivation and discipline.

But it is very interesting at the same time to make your routine very flexible. It should suit your conveniences. I can bet you that it is really not possible to workout at the same time of the day, every day. And also, it is not possible to have a daily 1 hour grinding for whatever real reasons we may face. So, you should be mentally prepared to have all these things incorporated in your regime. There are lots of sample workout routines you will see around the web by the experts on this field. But it is not mandatory that you should follow all these to master your workout, sometimes you will find contradictory as well. Also, I want to point one major thing for all of you here. We can have a minimum of 15 mins to maximum of 1 hour available in a day to do some workouts. In my opinion, spending an hour for your workout is more than sufficient for us to stay healthy. Remember, the quality is important above all. Just by staying at gym for 2 hours is not going to help you, if you just waste 30-45 mins there surfing your mobile and roaming around it. So given the time crunch we have, we should be very much focused on that much time we spend doing workouts. Before training your body, it is very much important to train your mind first. So, in summary all I want to say is, you should make your routine yourself just by experiencing few weeks of workout on your own. You give some time thinking about that when you are not doing anything, sitting idle at your couch.

In this chapter I am going to show you how you can manage your workout when you have 15 mins or 30 mins or 45 mins to 1 hour time with you. Because each day may be different for you handling various things. But doing a bare minimum on those time window will make you habituated. That is only going to make you consistent. I firmly believe that this mindset will help you to manage things in other aspect of your life as well. I have created two tables, one with having an access to your gym or weights and the other without having any access to a gym or having very minimal equipment handy at your home.

a. <u>Having access to GYM or major equipment</u>:

Workout Muscles	Total time			Starting after Long lag
	45mins-1hr	30 mins	10-15 mins	
Arms	**Triceps:** 1. Skull crusher 2. Rope pushdown 3. Overhead triceps extension by rope 4. Seated dips (finisher) **Biceps:** 5. Bicep curls (dumbbell and/or bar) 6. Hammer curls 7. Preacher curl 8. Rope curls (finisher)	You can remove one of the exercises in each category. And try super setting. **Triceps:** 1. Skull crusher 2. Rope pushdown 3. Overhead triceps extension by rope 4. Seated dips (finisher) **Biceps:** 5. Bicep curls (dumbbell and/or bar) 6. Hammer curls 7. Preacher curl 8. Rope curls (finisher)	Do these workouts in super sets. 1. a. rope pushdown b. rope biceps curl 2. a. overhead triceps extension b. hammer curls	Do only couple of exercises from each of triceps and biceps set. Also, the weight should be 50-60% of your max capacity.

#Bahubali

	45mins-1hr	30 mins	10-15 mins	Starting after Long lag
Chest	2. Pushups(warmup) 3. Barbell/dumbbell incline chest press. 4. Barbell/dumbbell flat chest press. 5. Barbell/Dumbbell decline chest press. 6. Butterfly 7. Cable crossover. 8. Chest dips	2. Pushups(warmup) 3. Barbell/dumbbell incline chest press. 4. Barbell/dumbbell flat chest press. 5. Chest dips. 6. butterfly	2. barbell/dumbbell incline chest press 3. chest dips 4. butterfly (if possible one set)	Do any two press workouts with 50-60% of your capacity. Do only pushups may be.
Legs	5. Regular squat 6. Leg press 7. Calf extension 8. Seated leg extension	4. Regular squat 5. Leg press 6. Calf extension	3. Regular squat 4. Calf extension	Incorporate very light squats and any other exercise from the list.
Back	6. Pull up 7. Deadlift 8. Lat pull down 9. Seated row 10. Single handed dumbbell row	6. Pull up 7. Deadlift 8. Lat pull down 9. Seated row 10. Straight arm rope pulldown (if permits only 1 failure set)	4. Pull up 5. Lat pull down 6. Straight arm rope pull down	3. Pull up 4. Any other listed exercise from the list apart from deadlift.

#BiggieMuscles

Shoulder	1. Military standing barbell press/seated dumbbell military press.
	 2. Dumbbell front raise.
	 3. Dumbbell/rope side raises.
	 4. Rope face pull.
	 5. Front plate raise/single arm lateral raise with dumbbell or rope.
		1. Military standing barbell press/seated dumbbell military press.
		 2. Dumbbell/rope side raises.
		 3. Rope face pull.
		 4. Front plate raise.
			1. Standing military press/ seated dumbbell military press.
			 2.
			   a. Dumbbell side raise.
			   b. Rope face pull
			 Do the exercises in 2, as supersets.
				1. Military press.
				 2. Lateral raise.
				 Do these exercises with 50-60% of your max capacity.

Abs	Do any 3 workouts comprising the upper abs, lower abs and obliques. But please note there is no meaning of doing countless ab exercises unless we follow a good diet. So, both of these go together to make your abs visible.			

#BoulderBeautiful

I have just given an overview of a sample workout routine which I preferably follow. Now it is your choice whether you will strictly follow this routine or create your own routine. The idea is to follow one, so that it becomes a habit and then stick to it. If you notice I have created 4 columns which pretty much covers the scenarios we face in our everyday life. When the time is less, I tried to give the workouts in such way so that it consists of entire part of the particular muscles. To elaborate more, when somedays the time is very less for you, try adding supersets/ drop sets in your regime. In case you are wondering what drop set is all about (most of you might be knowing already), it is having back-to-back sets with drop in weights in each set. So, these types of workouts will give you more intensity in a short workout window. This is what we all want to maximize the efficiency. So, if you go by this way, you will stay afloat in your goals whatever is the hindrance you face. Basically, there may be more than one exercise for the same part of the muscle on a given day, so when you are very tight on your time you may drop one of them and just go for another part of that muscle group. This helps in the completeness for the session in better way.

Yeah, there will be some phase where you have to miss continuous days of hitting the gym. And then once you come back you may feel low or may not. But the supreme idea is to restart it slowly. The world is not going to end if you are not able to lift the same weight (you used to lift few weeks back). So, for that I have made the last column in the table. You can customize it according to your own convenience. One more thing can happen is you are unable to hit the gym in person for some struggle but you can still manage somehow at your home, say during weekends. So, for that you might follow the next table which I have created for people having no access to gym or very minimal equipment at home. What I am trying to convey you is to find a way to do it.

Spend some of your spare time to think how you can create your own routine that may suit you the best. I only gave few exercises for each muscle group and there are hundreds more available. I only mentioned very important and efficient ones which you must do in order to grow. In case where you have shortage of any equipment at your gym, you may adjust with similar exercise one. So, you list out your own checking them over the internet.

In the above table one thing you might have noticed is, for abs exercises I didn't mention separately on different time management categories. This is because abs exercise you can also do at home in case it doesn't fit in your regular workout timings. It is always recommended to club the abs routines with any of your regular muscle workouts. In fact, it is not necessary that you do one muscle workout in each day. If you can afford having 5 days of regularity in your routine then you can go for it otherwise you can club one large muscle and one small muscle groups n the same day like chest/triceps, back/biceps etc. It is up to you how you decorate your routine over the week. Also, not every day you are going to spend the same amount of time at gym, in those scenarios all those time management workout routines I explained above, may come handy. You also need to keep in your mind that it is better to avoid workouts of same muscle categories within 24-48 hours. Because it is the recovery that is very much needed to build muscles, in the gym you just made the muscle work. I would suggest to have a minimum of 3 day and maximum of 5 days workout week. So accordingly, you create your own routine and follow. In the internet there are lot of weekly routines there, you are free to choose any of them which is suitable for you. If you ask me for preference, I will just tell you to follow bodybuilding.com website as they are very pro in this business and followed by billions of people.

b. <u>Having no access to GYM (or rather home type workout)</u>: Before I jump into the home workouts varieties, I would like to add few things about the potential constraints and requirements for home exercises. If your goal is to look toned or build/maintain muscle then I would definitely suggest you to have few home gears handy with you. Buy one pair of dumbbell or adjustable dumbbell which will suit across most workouts, or a pair of kettlebell or few resistance bands and start with that. This is on my personal experience as it helped me a lot during the lockdown phase. Also, to be honest, once you master the art of efficiency in doing home workouts, you will really feel very flexible for the days/weeks you unable to hit your regular gym destinations. It will also seem very helpful when someone is recovering from some injuries or coming out of some illness. So overall I very much value the home workout routines as par with outdoor gym workouts.

Work out Muscles	Total time			Starting after Long lag
	45mins-1hr	30 mins	10-15 mins	
Arms	1. a) dumbbell/band curls. b) overhead dumbbell/band extensions. 2. a) dumbbell/band hammer curls. b) triceps extensions with dumbbells/bands tied on a hinge. 3. a) seated single hand preacher curl. b) Lying French press. 4. a) overhand grip curl. b) triceps dips.	1. a) dumbbell/band curls. b) overhead dumbbell/band extensions. 2. a) dumbbell/band hammer curls. b) triceps extensions with dumbbells/bands tied on a hinge. 3. a) seated single hand preacher curl. b) triceps dips.	1. a) dumbbell/band curls. b) overhead dumbbell/band extensions. 2. a) dumbbell/band hammer curls. b) triceps extensions with dumbbells/bands tied on a hinge.	Do bodyweight triceps dips along with biceps curls (band or dumbbell) with max 10 reps.

#Gunnns

Chest	1. a) Incline/Flat pushups. b) Decline Pushups. 2. a) Floor dumbbell press. b) Door hinged resistance band chest fly. 3. a) Close grip Dumbbell squeeze press (for inner chest) b) Dumbbell chest fly. 4. Finisher low to high resistance band incline chest press. (As many reps as you can) + Dumbbell chest cross over (its across body and better to do it kneeled on the floor for max contraction)	1. a) Incline/Flat pushups. b) Decline Pushups. 2. a) Floor dumbbell press. b) Door hinged resistance band chest fly. 3. a) Close grip Dumbbell squeeze press (for inner chest) b) Dumbbell chest fly. Or, Any of the finisher movement in previous segment.	1. a) Incline/Flat pushups. b) Decline Pushups. 2. a) Close grip Dumbbell squeeze press (for inner chest) b) Dumbbell/banded chest fly. Do one set finisher if time permits.	Just do few pushups from different angle. May incorporate the banded chest flies.

#Chiseled

Legs				
Legs	1. Dumbbell/ Kettlebell squats (keeping them between legs) 2. Dumbbell lunges 3. Wall sits. (Start with holding for min 20-30 secs) 4. Alternate legs continuous reverse lunges. 5. Calf raises (support on a wall).	1. Dumbbell /Kettlebel l squats (keeping them between legs) 2. Dumbbell lunges. 3. Alternate legs continuou s reverse lunges. 4. Calf raises (support on a wall).	1. Dumbbel l/Kettleb ell squats (keeping them between legs) 2. DB lunges.	Do only the squats and reverse lunges with max 10 reps in each set.

#ShakeYourLeg

Back				
Back	1. Pull up (if some high hinge available at home) 2. Dumbbell single hand row. 3. Row with resistance band (hinged at the door) 4. Lat pull down with resistance band. 5. Back extension with a towel.	1. Pull up (if some high hinge available at home) 2. Dumbbell single hand row. 3. Row with resistance band (hinged at the door) 4. Lat pull down with resistance band. or Back extension with a towel.	1. Dumbbell single hand row. 2. Row with resistance band (hinged at the door)	Do the row exercises with DB or Resistance bands.

#V-taper

Shoulder	1. DB shoulder press. 2. DB front raise. 3. DB lateral raise. 4. A. Resistance band slow front raise. B. resistance band lateral raise.	1. DB shoulder press. 2. DB front raise. 3. DB lateral raise.	1. DB shoulder press. 2. DB lateral raise.	Do 3-4 sets of shoulder press and lateral raise combined.

#FrontLoad

So, as you have seen I tried to add mostly some superset type of exercises for home workouts. since you have minimal equipment at home, you need to make sure that the intensity will be high to make up to some extent. Do the supersets, giant set (if you don't know already, it is combination of 3 back-to-back exercises), drop sets for your home workout tricks and maximize the work being put on.

For the rep-ranges I will suggest to keep it between 12-20. If you are going to have only a pair of dumbbells then just go for the optimum one which will help you do most of the exercises as per your level. Bands are cheaper in that sense, so you can go for it with multiple strengths. These will help you to cover the weight ranges of your exercises.

As another trick, sometimes go super slow for the last few reps (3-5) in the negatives. This will help you feel the actual light weight heavier and increase the tension. Remember it's the constant tension that helps the muscles to grow. So, you need to constantly spice up and innovate things to get the maximum benefits. For an example you can just count 1-5 while going slow in your negatives.

- **Stretching/Warm-ups:**

So, earlier I had mentioned about different workout moves and routines that you can follow in your bodybuilding process. One very important lesson also I have learnt over the years is to incorporate different kind of stretching movement in your workout. These are very essential to have an injury free phase during your workout time which ultimately paves the way to have better longevity to continue your grind. Before and after each workout session, if you are doing heavy weight training it is recommended to have a very little amount of stretching of your muscles. Stretching helps the muscles to get accustomed with the load of work you are going to put on them over next few minutes. It helps people to get more flexible and focused while completing the entire workout session. This in turn prevent any serious injury. It also helps in getting good recovery between the sets. Post workout stretches helps you to get rid of the soreness, improve blood flow, move lactic acids out of the muscle and so forth.

Even for people who are comfortable with doing only bodyweight exercises, they can do the stretching of full body to get more of a feel at the start of their session. See, all these little things are very paramount to have a very satisfying session for the day. So let us not ignore it any time and always try to keep this in mind.

In the context of this book, I also thought of the condition of people like us who work behind the desk for most part of the day in their professional lives. We cannot deny the super annoying back pain we get very often these days. So, I am very much proponent of the fact that even in the days when we are not doing any special workout session, we must need to do some kind of stretching moves to get rid of that stiffness at least. I have given few stretching moves in this chapter that can help you to feel well from the blues of daily work.

A. *Stretching moves for pre & post workouts:*

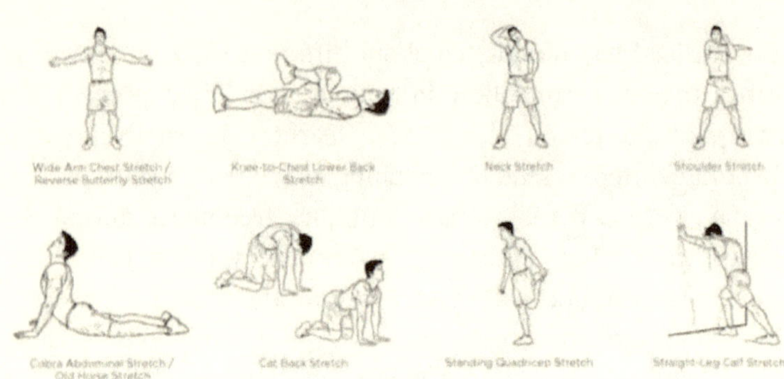

#stretching

These are some common stretching exercises we can do pre and post of our workout. Mostly it is preferable to do some dynamic stretches for pre-workout like arm circles, butt kicks etc. and to do some static stretches for post-workout like shoulder stretch, butterfly stretch etc.

B. *Stretching moves to get rid of back stiffness:*

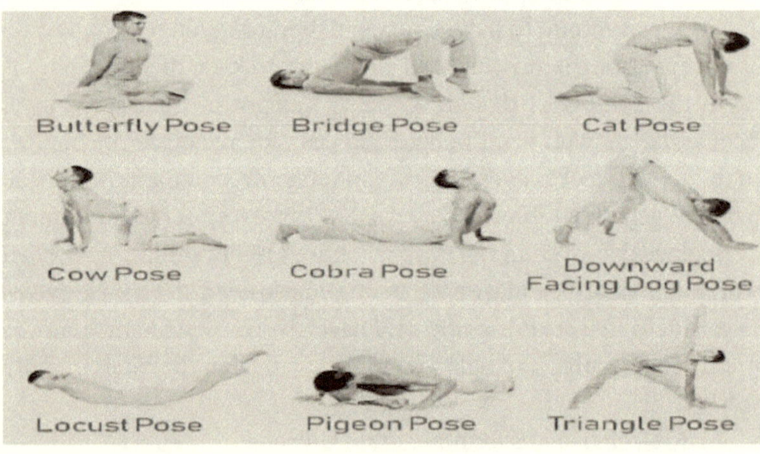

#ByeByeBackStiffness

C. Stretching moves at your desk:

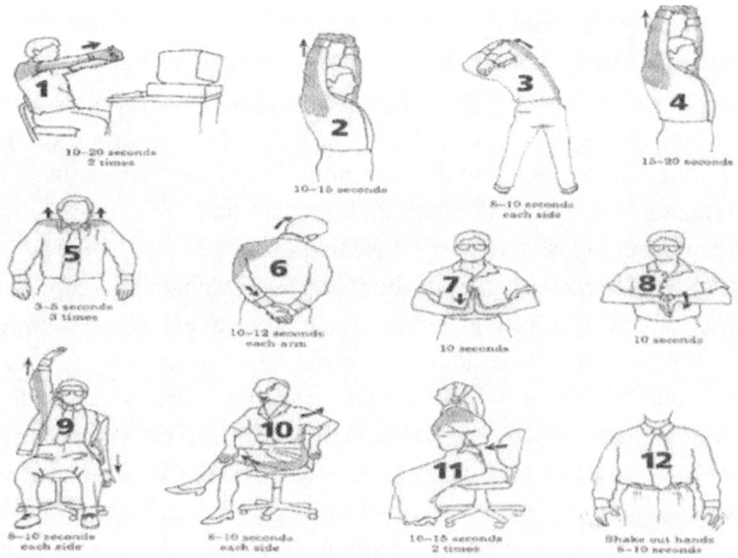

#Fun@work

- **Yoga:**

You may be wondering what is the context of yoga here since I have mostly covered the typical muscle building practices throughout this chapter. Well, yoga has its own aura in the fitness culture. People who are very immersed in the bodybuilding workout habits, may not like this topic much but after this short discussion you will understand how the yoga can help you to perform in better level in your upcoming days. Sometimes you may feel very bored and may lack that focus in your normal workout days. And as we all know we need to do something different to get back the rhythm and enthusiasm. It is needless to say that yoga might help you in this scenario as I am telling you from my very own experiences. You will feel more rejuvenation in your original routine for sure. Even, the yoga moves give us the advantages to build great flexibility, stamina and strength.

I highly recommend that you must try the yoga in your fitness journey either when you face the aforementioned situation or you want to experiment with something new without compromising the activeness in your lifestyle. Also, there is one important reason to touch upon this topic is, sometimes people face some life changing injuries in their lives and they are unable to continue the weight training exercises they love to do. In those cases, may be for years while recovering from the injury, it is obvious to keep away from any weight lifting moves. Some well guided yoga routines always help as some kind of rehab. One more way, we can incorporate yoga is when you feel that the progress has stalled for some time. Then you can switch to any efficient yoga routine on your own and then come back after a month to your original workout regime.

For people who can keep minimum 15-20 mins daily or alternate days for their physical activities, a compact yoga routine is what they can always look for. I personally followed a 15 min yoga routine every alternate day when I was recovering from Covid, for a month and it really did wonders for me. You might be well following the yoga for rest of your life and that will give you a tremendous advantage of maintaining good health over long period of time. And more importantly you don't need to spend much also for equipment, only a good yoga mat pretty much is needed as your companion.

"If you have discipline, drive, determination, nothing is impossible." **– Dana Linn Bailey, First Ever Women's Physique Olympia Champion.**

CHAPTER FOUR

THE COMMON DISCIPLINED DIET & ADDONS...

As we reach into the end of this book, it is very obvious to say that whatever we have learnt thus far, cannot be completed successfully unless we follow the habit of quality food intake. I have heard a lot of time, be it in social media or any website from different experts that Diet is more important than the exercise. There is also a very famous quote you might have come across that "abs are made in kitchen". I am not against these concepts but I must say that there are very few experts I have seen talking and emphasizing on "100% diet and 100% exercise" criteria, which very much makes sense to me. You just cannot overweight either of your diet or the effort you put on workout. They produce magic only when they are followed with great discipline.

In this chapter I will not talk about any fancy diet charts, there are too many over the internet which you can check definitely but I doubt about the feasibility of them in longer term. You need not to be too strict upon yourselves for a certain period of time and then you just make up your food cravings so badly by eating junk food every other day after that. This will just undo all your hard work in few weeks, if not in few days. You are free to choose your own brand of food as long as they are pretty clean in terms of quality.

It's up to you, how you distribute your foods over the day as you might remember the equation I spoke about earlier, it is all about the calorie intake and burning. Every one of us have grown up in different places with different set of food choices. But I promise you, each one of us have our own set of healthy foods in our respective cultures, you just need to devote sometime to shortlist them (in case you haven't already ?).

Another important point I want to highlight here is that, sometime you may see many bodybuilders put their pics with lot of burgers, wings, fries etc. in the social media. You may find it very disturbing and confusing actually. No, they can't just maintain a body eating those junk foods to be honest. I have seen few of them only showing these types of pics every week but don't show the good quality foods which people should take. So, don't believe on those bullshit if you are one still confused. But at the same time, I also need to mention, that eating a junk food once in a while doesn't make you sinner nonetheless. Basically, both of the types of myth go around us when it comes to diet, so it is my first job to make you people very clear on this.

You should always maintain a diet that is helpful for you in long term. I don't think each one of us is comfortable in taking foods which are only boiled, foods without salt/sugar etc. day in day out. All micro/macro ingredients have their own good sides in our body composition. You can definitely take sugar in certain amount if you are finding it difficult without it. The cravings should not be such that you overeat in few days and let your hard work gets the injustice.

So, here I am going to show you a food chart that I normally follow happily and also mention some suggestions as alternatives too. You can replace the components with something that fits your choice which obviously needs to be clean in its calorific values and quality. I am a non veg by birth but I have mentioned the foods from veg categories as well. Don't just think that you cannot build your dream physique if you are veg, there are lot of well-known personalities out there who are veg and at the same time they pose great physiques which can be envied of.

Breakfast	Late morning	Lunch	Snacks	Post workout	Dinner
Quaker oats with skimmed milk, 2-4 egg whites/protein banana pancakes	Few almonds, dates, coffee/tea	Rice+sabji+fish /chicken/egg/paner Curry + salad	1 banana/apple + coffee/tea (15-20 mins before workout)	Protein shake + 1 banana + 5-10 egg whites	Rice/chapati sabji+fish /chicken/egg/paner Curry + salad

#YumYum

As you see this routine is very much customized for me and I myself organized it as per my convenience. I mostly (~99% of time) do my workouts at the evening right after my office hours, so I have managed the food timings in that way. If some of you are comfortable with early morning workouts then please go ahead and tweak this routine a little bit like you may have breakfast right after your morning workout and you can add one banana onto it, then you can add the eggs either before lunch or in the evening time between snacks and dinner. Other than the big 3 meals, whenever you are going for some snacks be it in afternoon or in the morning, try to have healthy options like some nuts, yogurts etc. You can add yogurt/dahi with your lunch/dinner as well.

I like to have oats in the morning for most of the days, but when I feel a little bored then I opt for multigrain bread toasts or I prepare protein pancakes (checkout my Instagram handle for my handmade pancakes and ingredients :)). Besides as a replacement you can try idly or chapati (as most Indian households are habituated to) in the breakfast. Just find your right food and hold onto that. You mix that up over the weeks so that you don't get too bored.

In the lunch and dinner, you may have noticed I always have some non veg curry or sometime paneer curry. Along with that I prefer to have a sabji which I mostly try to be protein rich like rajma, soyabean, palak etc. You might also have observed that I haven't very definitive about calorie calculations here but I am also not too careless here. I add some kind of salad just to fill my stomach so that I don't overeat the rice or chapatis. Someday you may not feel having salads also, and that is absolutely ok. You can have carrots, cucumber, lettuce etc. as part of the salad, just don't think you need to bite some fancy leaves otherwise you are done. There is nothing like that and don't believe on people also who tells that.

Supplements: If I don't tell anything about the supplements then you probably think that I am hiding it from you. Well, it is very much true that if you are really going to put on some visible muscle then you have to take care of your daily protein intake. Possibly for skinny guys who are going to start bodybuilding, they will get hard times while putting on some serious muscle. You need to maintain your protein intake to some surplus quantity. "Most" of the times we don't find that adequate amount of protein in our daily food intake given our current lifestyle. So, in that case it is obvious that you need to look for some protein supplements (specifically Whey protein) which suits your body. It is very important to understand here that the protein supplement you are going to stick upon must be authentic and also it should suit your digestion. From my personal experience I must tell you not all whey protein products are going to work for you. I don't want to recommend any special brand here, it's on you to decide after doing some basic research. Don't always look for any cheap alternative in this case as it may hinder your progress and you might also develop some side effects. So, you need to be very cautious on this choice. If you ask me, I generally prefer using whey protein from the brand ON (optimum nutrition) given its proven quality over the years and reviews. But again, I encourage you to do your own research and experiment on you and then stick to it. Beware of the authenticity of the product as well when you are buying online. You don't want to risk your health here while trying to improve your result. At the same time, you also need to ensure you are drinking enough water (3-4 ltr) throughout the day. Do remember one thing, if you are getting enough protein from your daily food intake its absolutely makes sense not to go for any supplement also. Trust me, I have seen one of my colleagues having nice muscular physique without any whey protein supplement. There is no replacement of whole foods for the basic nutrients you need when it is cooked properly.

Now protein is one part of the supplement, there are other supplements also available which bodybuilders try out. There are vitamins, fish oil, BCAA, glutamine, creatine and so on. But trust me, you don't need any of these if you are having a very balanced diet in your lifestyle. Also, if someone has just started bodybuilding then it is highly recommended that you don't need to depend on these for initial years. Let's say if you are having hard time between strenuous workouts for some time due to some reason (not enough energy leading to workout), you can opt for having BCAA solution between workouts. but it is obvious to say, don't stick on these things for long time unless you are guided by any certified trainer or so. I really want you people to dig more on these things in the internet, learn from some best-known experts around the world and take decision. I have seen folks who just believe that taking these supplements is the key but don't do workout correctly in the gym. Don't just trust the sayings, you are the better judge here. The more convincing you become, the easier it becomes.

- **Few Interesting Recipes (at your convenience):**

In this section I am going to give some useful details of healthy recipes that you can always try at your home. I personally have this very often just to make my everyday diet interesting enough.

i. *Banana Protein Pancake*:

Ingredients:
1 banana, 2 egg whites/whole, 1 scoop protein powder, handful oats(optional), baking soda(optional).

Procedure:

- Keep your mixer/grinder clean and put 1 large banana cut into slices in it.
- Add 2 egg whites or whole eggs breaking into it, this will provide the liquid for the mixture. So, when you are going to make a large number of pancakes, make sure to add more eggs into it to increase the liquid proportion of the final batter. Don't add water into it to increase the liquid as it causes problem during cooking in the pan later.
- Add 1 scoop of protein powder into it along with a palmful of oats on top of it. If anyone doesn't have the protein powder then they can go for some whole wheat/corn flour to replace that. For the sake of the name of this recipe I preferred protein powder to be added here. You can add baking soda also to have more fluffiness of the pancakes, but this is optional. Now grind the mixture in a blender to get the batter.
- Now pre-heat the pan, add very little healthy oil (I prefer olive oil) into it and just spread it. You can use a cooking spray as well or use a brush to soak the entire pan with little oil.
- Now from the container, pour the amount of batter into the pan to have medium/standard sized pancake. You cook for 3-5 mins one side and the moment you see most of the holes has popped up from the half-cooked batter just flip it. Then cook for another 3-5 mins and you are done with 1 delicious pancake. Finish your batter and enjoy your breakfast.
- You can eat with little honey or some peanut butter if you wish. But please don't put any sugar/jaggery with the mixture as the pancake will come out as sweetened already.

i. **Medium Spicy and healthy chicken curry:**

Ingredients: Chicken curry cut, onion, curd/yogurt, tomato, garam masala

Procedure:

- Marinade the chicken pieces with curd, turmeric powder and salt, well before the cooking time.
- Add 2-3 spoon of oil into the cooking pan and then pour the onion pieces (2-3 medium sized onion) and tomato pieces along with the whole. Then stir it for sometime until the orange tomato mix becomes golden brown. Do this in medium flame.
- After that add the marinaded chicken mixture into the pan and stir well until the spices gets evenly mixed with the chicken pieces. Add a cover and cook it in slow flames for 40-45 mins.

iii. **Mexican burrito meal:**

Ingredients: Rajma, boiled rice, chicken breast (for veg just replace it with paneer/tofu), tomato, capsicum, salsa, barbeque or tomato sauce, sweet corn.
Procedure:

- Have your rajma and rice boiled already before the actual mixture to be prepared.
- The chicken breast should be marinated at least 3-4 hours before it is being cooked, keeping it for overnight may be best. For marination, pour some good quality oil in small quantity, then add cumin powder, garlic-ginger powder, paprika, barbeque sauce, salt as per taste, oregano mixture. You can add some chat masala as well for enhanced spicy feel as per your wish. The chicken breast size should be kept medium as you got normally from the shop.
- Cut the tomato, capsicum, salsa in small pieces.
- Have the sweet corn sautéed with very minimal butter in the pan.
- Now for cooking the chicken, have a little amount of oil sprayed or spread in the pan. Then put the cut chicken breast into pan once the pan is heated in medium flame for some time. Let it be cooked for 5-7 mins and then you flip the other side and cook for same amount of time. After that put the cooked chicken breasts

into a plate, don't cut it into pieces immediately otherwise the juice will be gone.

- Now take a medium to large sized bowl and put the cut veggies, corn, rice and boiled rajma inside that. You can cut the cooked chicken breasts now after 7-10 mins into mini pieces and then add it into the bowl. You can add some lettuce also in the end on top of that and also you can add a little more sauce if you are fond of that. Now your burrito rice bowl is ready to be eaten. Enjoy your meal.

iv. **Grilled chicken steak meal:**

Ingredients: Chicken breast, veggies like capsicum, carrots, asparagus, marinated items like salt, pepper, cumin powder, paprika, ginger-garlic powder, 1-2 spoon of olive oil, lemon.
Procedure:

- Cut the chicken breasts to medium size. Then marinate it with little oil, salt, cumin powder, pepper, paprika, ginger-garlic powder. Don't forget to add the lemon squeezed juice, it generally helps your digestion.
- Keep the grilled pan or normal non sticky pan in the oven and heat for 2 mins and then pour/brush very little amount of olive oil there (we already gave oil during marination part, so this time very little oil is required). Put the chicken breasts one by one into the pan and cook one side for 5-7 mins in medium flame. Then once the sides are becoming white, flip them to cook other side for same amount of time. Once both sides are cooked, take it out into a plate and let it cool down for another 5 mins.
- You can sauté the vegetables in the pan leftover or you can have it cut raw and clean.
- Once you cut the chicken breast into parallel pieces, serve it with the vegetables. You can also add some mashed potato into it to get the restaurant feel.

- You can prepare this dish into micro-oven as well by setting it into grilled mode.
- **Tips**: before marinating, you can have little holes into the chicken breast pieces just to ensure the ingredients go into it nice and rich. Keeping it for overnight is the best you can do for the right taste.

v. Grilled Basa fish steak meal:

This recipe is pretty similar to the grilled chicken recipe I just elaborated earlier. Only you have to replace the chicken by the fish. The marination ingredients you can keep almost same, you can add any extra of your choice on your knowledge also. Otherwise, the process remains same.

vi. Grilled/roasted chicken drumsticks for snacks:

Ingredients: chicken drumsticks, 1-2 table spoon of oil, ginger garlic powder, cumin powder, paprika, chicken/chat masala (optional), Sauce of your choice, lemon.
Procedure:

- Get the pieces of chicken drumsticks marinated with little bit of oil, ginger garlic powder, cumin powder, paprika, salt, sauce of your choice (bbq or tomato) and lemon juice. You can add little bit of chicken masala or chat masala too if you want more spice and flavor. If you can brush the oil on all the pieces then it is better. Keep the mixture at least 3-4 hours before cooking.
- You can use microwave for this recipe or can be done in pan as well. For microwave you should put the settings into grill/combi (approx. 70-30 gill and roast) and let it cook for 20-25 mins on one side and then flip the other side to cook for 15-20 mins. In pan you should cook each side for 15-20 mins. Then you can serve it hot with any sauce of your choice with few slices of onion.

vii.   **Lightly oven fried chickpeas for snacks:**

Ingredients: Dry Soaked chickpeas, finely chopped onions, sliced tomato, little around 1 table spoon oil, cumin powder.
Procedure:

- Keep the chickpeas in water overnight. Then just before cooking dry it out completely.
- In a pan apply very little oil (or spray cooking oil) in medium heat. Then add the cumin powder (or you can use whole jeera as well), chopped onion and tomatoes onto it. Optionally you can add sliced/whole green chilly as well. Green chilly will give you the flavor.
- Now within 2-3 mins add the dried chickpeas into the pan. Stir the entire mixture now for some time like 5-10 mins.
- Once done you can sprinkle few seasonings or chat masala in small quantities and then enjoy your food.

viii.   **Healthy chicken sandwich:**

Ingredients: Sandwich/multigrain/brown bread slices, boneless chicken fillet or breast, chopped onion, ginger, tomatoes, cumin powder, turmeric powder, salt, seasonings.
Process:

- Marinate the boneless chicken with salt, cumin powder, turmeric powder and with your choice of seasonings. Keep it for at least 3-4 hours prior to the preparation. Don't cut the chicken into small pieces initially. You do it later and that makes it tastier.
- Now apply 1-2 table spoon of oil into the pan into medium heat. Then put the chopped onions, ginger and tomatoes into it. After that put the pieces of chicken into it. Cook each side for 5-10 mins. Once the cooking is done for both sides keep the chicken as it is for 2-5 mins more into the plate.

- Cut the cooked chicken now into very small pieces. Now between two pieces of the breads keep the cut chicken. You can put the breads now within a sandwich maker or you can heat it into the pan for 5-7 mins for each side of the bread.
- Please avoid mayonnaise or cheese in this recipe otherwise the healthiness quotient will not matter much.
- You can add cut cucumber in your sandwich also at the end if you want.

ix. **Sweet corn and soya sandwich:**

Ingredients: Whole wheat or brown bread, Soya chunks, sweet corn, cumin whole, carrot, cucumber; optional (potato, lettuce, tomato)

Process:

- Boil the soya chunks and then let it dry. If you have bigger chunks then cut it into small pieces, small soya chunks are preferred.
- Boil the sweet corns also and optionally you can stir it in the pan with very little butter.
- Now boil the potato and get it mashed.
- In the frying pan with medium heat, stir the cumin seeds for 1-2 mins. Then add the cumin into the mashed potato along with the soya chunks and sweet corns. Mix them well and add the salt as per taste. You can add green chilly also into the mixture.
- Then you should be ready with the bread being toasted and then put the mixture inside the slices along with some fresh carrots being grated, and cucumber slices. There is also one other way to do this if you have sandwich maker. First put the mixture within the slices and then make it toasted inside the machine. Now your sandwich is ready to be served and enjoy this delicious snack.

If you are looking for less calorie then just remove the potato from the recipe and that's all.

I have given you few easy to cook recipes so far. You can add these in your food habit at your own conveniences. You might have realized that these recipes also take very less time which might help you in your busy schedule to adjust but not compromising with your fitness journey. Just want to mention that the time given in the procedure of above recipes is approximate ones. Don't be disheartened if you fail at your first attempt. Once you make it as a habit you will master this art too. Specially the snacks mentioned in the list are very good alternative to any outside junk food. During the afternoon or evening time we all crave for some snacks and most of the times I have found out the options around me is relatively unhealthy. If you are the person who wants to have snacks around that time, I will say you can go for having a mixture of makhana and almonds. Makhana is very protein rich in nature and tasty at the same time. I am very thankful to my mother for this great food idea which she prepared one day and after that it has become my go to option whenever I have the crave to eat some snack around my evening workout time or even in a rest day.

I also promise that these recipes are seriously tasty enough. I wanted to emphasize on this fact because most people believe that health foods are bound to be tasteless. So, I would suggest just try these in your own hand and break the myth at your ease.

Also, you can add your own masala into these recipes to get your type flavor, just be careful of not adding too much unhealthy stuffs. As you see it's not that tough here to follow a diet. It is good to customize your own way as long as it stays healthy enough for you. There is no point to be overwhelmed or confused over the jargons of fitness diets that goes around us every day everywhere.

"Healthy eating is a way of life, so it's important to establish routines that are simple, realistically, and ultimately livable." – **Horace**

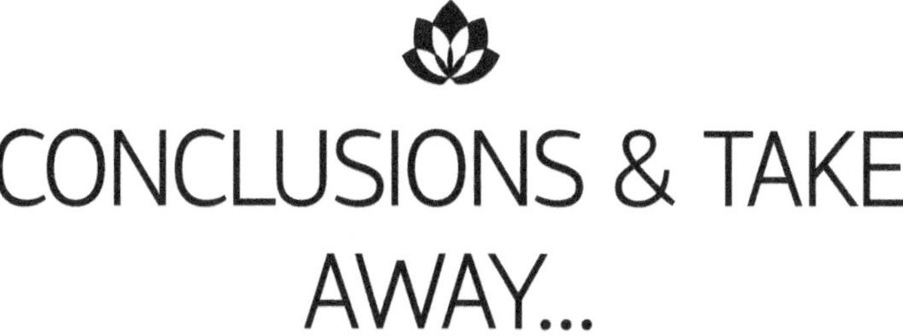

CHAPTER FIVE

CONCLUSIONS & TAKE AWAY...

So, you have just completed this book with all the tips and tricks I wanted to share with all of you. I hope I am able to present the right ways on your goal to build a decent physique. As you observed already, I have tried to tell one thing again and again and that is **discipline**. After a certain point the so called 'motivation' may not work and that's why you need to think beyond it. Everyday 20 mins can do wonders for you if you are doing the right way rather than just giving up after 1 month. I am encouraging you to make your own routine as per your conveniences. Take help from what is there in the internet and create your own regime. Set very practical and feasible goals every day/month/year. Always think you are different and we have our barriers obviously, so don't compare yours with others out there. Try to be very patient in this game, when you see the results that's when you will surely be going to be motivated more. So, wait for that minimum time my friend. Also, I must say that always apply logic in whatever way you are following your goals. You just cannot keep following a low carb diet for your lifetime so be very clear about that. There are lot of such "sayings/ mantras" out there which you need to accept or reject with clarity. Don't be too paranoid also regarding your habits like someday you might miss something. If you get stressed on something that helps you to get out of everyday stress, then that is not going to help you at all. So, take it easy and don't give up.

Summarizing all the above factors together with consistent good sleep will definitely aid your progress, so you definitely need to take care of that as well. Always try to maintain a good sound sleeping habits of at least 6-8 hours daily. If you exercise hard daily but deprive yourself of sleep, you may even see some health issues. Without a good sleep from previous night, you will not get the right amount energy to do some workout sessions. I know you might have seen people showing off in the social media talking about how hard they are pushing themselves in the gym even though they are having very small amount of sleep. But trust me, you don't need to compare your case with themselves. Its just absolutely scientific that workout, good food habits and so daily good sleep cycle all together will give you the perfect ingredients to achieve your fitness goals.

I think I have done my part through this book to show you a path how to do it. Now it's time for you to just believe in this and move on. Feel free to share your progress or feedback to me any time in my email mentioned below. I am very eager to know and interact with you people how you feel about this little guidance I tried to log with all my limited experiences. I wish you all success in all the field and looking forward to talk to you.

***"If I can see it and believe it, then I can achieve it."* – Arnold Schwarzenegger, One of the greatest bodybuilder of all time.**

Email: meranaamjoker1221@gmail.com

Linked-In: https://www.linkedin.com/in/sandipan-haldar-24244716/

Instagram: sandipanhaldar